A Heartfelt Thank You!

As the author of this book, I am deeply grateful for your support and readership. If you've enjoyed the journey through the pages, please consider sharing your thoughts with a review on Amazon. Your feedback not only helps us to improve but also guides fellow readers. Thank you for being a part of our story!

Table of Contents

Introduction

Welcome to a nostalgic journey through the vibrant eras of the 1950s to the 1990s—a time of remarkable change and cultural milestones. This trivia book is a treasure trove of memories for the Baby Boomer generation and beyond, inviting you to relive the iconic moments in music, cinema, sports, history, science, and inventions that defined these dynamic decades.

Each page is filled with carefully crafted questions that will challenge your knowledge and rekindle the spirit of times when vinyl ruled the music scene, classic films captured our hearts, sporting legends were made, and groundbreaking inventions reshaped our world.

Whether you're a trivia enthusiast, a history buff, or simply looking to reminisce, this collection is your ticket to the past. It's more than just a quiz; it's a celebration of the moments that have brought us to where we are today. So, gather your friends, test your wits, and enjoy the ride through the golden years of the 20th century.

Let the trivia begin!

How to Use This Trivia Book

Here's how to get the most out of your experience:

1. **Dive into Each Section**: The book is organized by decades and topics—Music, Cinema, Sport, History, Science, and Inventions. Start from the beginning or jump to your favorite era or subject.

2. **Engage with the Questions**: Each question is designed to be thought-provoking and fun. Read them aloud, ponder, and guess before you check the answers.

3. **Check Your Answers**: Once you've given your best shot at the questions, turn to the last page of the book where all the correct answers are listed for easy verification.

4. **Make It Social**: Challenge friends and family to a trivia night, or use the questions to spark conversations and share memories.

5. **Enjoy the Nostalgia**: Whether you're right or wrong, each question is an opportunity to reminisce about the good old days.

Remember, there's no timer here. Take your time, enjoy the trivia, and let the good times roll!

Happy reminiscing!

The 1950's

The Fabulous 1950s: A Decade of Transformation and Triumph

Step into the 1950s, a decade where post-war prosperity gave rise to a cultural revolution that still resonates today. It was a time of optimism, where innovation met with the rhythm of rock 'n' roll, and the silver screen sparkled with Technicolor dreams.

This was the era of the American Dream, where suburbs grew, cars were king, and televisions became the hearth of every home. The '50s saw the birth of youth culture, the civil rights movement began to stir, and the space race took our eyes to the stars.

As you embark on this section of trivia, prepare to be whisked back to the days of Elvis Presley's swiveling hips, Marilyn Monroe's dazzling charm, and the first whispers of a digital revolution. The 1950s were a time to rebuild, reinvent, and rejoice.

Let's see how much you remember from this iconic decade!

1. *Who released the hit song "Heartbreak Hotel" in 1956?*

A	Chuck Berry	B	Elvis Presley
C	Jerry Lee Lewis	D	Buddy Holly

2. *What genre of music became popular in the 1950s?*

A	Disco	B	Rock 'n' Roll
C	Jazz	D	Blues

3. *Which female artist was known as the "Queen of Rock 'n' Roll" in the 1950s?*

A	Patsy Cline	B	Billie Holiday
C	Ella Fitzgerald	D	Wanda Jackson

4. *"The Day the Music Died" refers to the death of which musician?*

A	Elvis Presley	B	Ritchie Valens
C	Buddy Holly	D	Chuck Berry

5. *Which 1950s dance was named after a city in South Carolina?*

A	Twist	B	Jitterbug
C	Charleston	D	Mambo

6. *Which song by Bill Haley & His Comets is considered one of the first rock and roll records?*

A	Rock Around the Clock	B	Tutti Frutti
C	Hound Dog	D	Jailhouse Rock

7. *Who was nicknamed 'The King of Swing'?*

A	Louis Armstrong	B	Benny Goodman
C	Duke Ellington	D	Glenn Miller

8. *What was the name of Elvis Presley's debut album?*

A	Blue Suede Shoes	B	Elvis Presley
C	Love Me Tender	D	Heartbreak Hotel

9. *Which 1950s hit begins with the line 'One, two, three o'clock, four o'clock rock'?*

A) Rock Around the Clock	B) Good Golly Miss Molly
C) Johnny B. Goode	D) Jailhouse Rock

10. *'La Bamba' is a traditional song made famous by which artist?*

A) Carlos Santana	B) Ritchie Valens
C) Desi Arnaz	D) Antonio Carlos Jobim

11. *Which artist is known for the hit "What'd I Say"?*

A) Ray Charles	B) Chuck Berry
C) Fats Domino	D) Little Richard

12. *"Mack the Knife" was a famous song by which singer?*

A) Frank Sinatra	B) Dean Martin
C) Bobby Darin	D) Sammy Davis Jr.

13. *Which group released "Sh-Boom" in 1954?*

A. The Platters

B. The Chords

C. The Drifters

D. The Coasters

14. *Who is credited with popularizing the electric guitar in the 1950s?*

A. Muddy Waters

B. B.B. King

C. Chuck Berry

D. Les Paul

15. *"Only You" was a hit for which vocal group?*

A. The Drifters

B. The Flamingos

C. The Platters

D. The Moonglows

16. *Which song by The Everly Brothers topped the charts in 1957?*

A. Bye Bye Love

B. Wake Up Little Susie

C. All I Have to Do Is Dream

D. Cathy's Clown

17. *"Great Balls of Fire" was a hit for which rock and roll artist?*

A. Elvis Presley
B. Jerry Lee Lewis
C. Little Richard
D. Chuck Berry

18. *What instrument is associated with Fats Domino?*

A. Guitar
B. Saxophone
C. Piano
D. Drums

19. *Who sang the classic song "Peggy Sue"?*

A. Buddy Holly
B. Roy Orbison
C. Gene Vincent
D. Eddie Cochran

20. *"Summertime Blues" was a 1958 hit for which artist?*

A. Chuck Berry
B. Eddie Cochran
C. Bo Diddley
D. Carl Perkins

21. *Which actor starred as 'Ricky Ricardo' in 'I Love Lucy'?*

A	Desi Arnaz	B	William Frawley
C	Vivian Vance	D	Fred MacMurray

22. *What was the first animated feature film to be nominated for an Oscar?*

A	Peter Pan	B	Lady and the Tramp
C	Cinderella	D	Sleeping Beauty

23. *Who directed the epic film 'Ben-Hur'?*

A	Cecil B. DeMille	B	William Wyler
C	Alfred Hitchcock	D	Orson Welles

24. *Which movie features the song 'Singing in the Rain'?*

A	An American in Paris	B	The Band Wagon
C	Singin' in the Rain	D	On the Town

25. *'The Twilight Zone' TV series was created by which individual?*

A	Alfred Hitchcock	B	Rod Serling
C	Gene Roddenberry	D	Orson Welles

26. *Which actress won an Oscar for 'Roman Holiday'?*

A	Audrey Hepburn	B	Grace Kelly
C	Elizabeth Taylor	D	Vivien Leigh

27. *What was the first color TV show broadcast by NBC?*

A	The Colgate Comedy Hour	B	Bonanza
C	The Rose Bowl	D	The Today Show

28. *Who hosted 'The $64,000 Question' game show?*

A	Groucho Marx	B	Hal March
C	Bob Barker	D	Jack Barry

29. *Which film featured Marilyn Monroe's iconic white dress scene?*

A Gentlemen Prefer Blondes

B How to Marry a Millionaire

C The Seven Year Itch

D Some Like It Hot

30. *'Gunsmoke' debuted on TV in what year?*

A 1950

B 1955

C 1957

D 1960

31. *Who played the lead role in 'The African Queen'?*

A Humphrey Bogart

B Clark Gable

C Cary Grant

D James Stewart

32. *Which TV show featured the character 'Lucy Ricardo'?*

A The Honeymooners

B Leave It to Beaver

C I Love Lucy

D Father Knows Best

33. *'On the Waterfront' won the Best Picture Oscar in which year?*

A. 1952	B. 1954
C. 1956	D. 1958

34. *Which actress is remembered for her role in 'Rear Window'?*

A. Audrey Hepburn	B. Grace Kelly
C. Ingrid Bergman	D. Elizabeth Taylor

35. *What was the popular children's show hosted by Bob Keeshan?*

A. The Mickey Mouse Club	B. Captain Kangaroo
C. Lassie	D. The Lone Ranger

36. *Which classic western series began in 1959?*

A. Bonanza	B. The Rifleman
C. Gunsmoke	D. Rawhide

37. *Who starred as 'Moses' in the 1956 film 'The Ten Commandments'?*

A. Charlton Heston
B. Yul Brynner
C. Kirk Douglas
D. Burt Lancaster

38. *What was the first film to be released in CinemaScope?*

A. The Robe
B. How to Marry a Millionaire
C. East of Eden
D. Rebel Without a Cause

39. *Which actress played opposite James Stewart in 'Vertigo'?*

A. Kim Novak
B. Janet Leigh
C. Grace Kelly
D. Eva Marie Saint

40. *'Father Knows Best' transitioned from radio to television in what year?*

A. 1951
B. 1954
C. 1956
D. 1958

41. *Who won the FIFA World Cup in 1954?*

A	Brazil	B	Italy
C	West Germany	D	Uruguay

42. *Which boxer was the World Heavyweight Champion from 1952 to 1956?*

A	Joe Louis	B	Rocky Marciano
C	Muhammad Ali	D	Floyd Patterson

43. *What major league baseball player hit 660 home runs?*

A	Babe Ruth	B	Hank Aaron
C	Willie Mays	D	Mickey Mantle

44. *Who set the hour record in cycling in 1954?*

A	Jacques Anquetil	B	Fausto Coppi
C	Eddy Merckx	D	Louison Bobet

45. *Which country hosted the 1956 Summer Olympics?*

A. United States

B. Soviet Union

C. Australia

D. Italy

46. *Which golfer won the Masters Tournament twice in the 1950s?*

A. Ben Hogan

B. Arnold Palmer

C. Gary Player

D. Sam Snead

47. *What was the nickname of New York Yankees legend Mickey Mantle?*

A. The Sultan of Swat

B. The Commerce Comet

C. Mr. October

D. The Iron Horse

48. *Who broke the four-minute mile in 1954?*

A. John Landy

B. Glenn Cunningham

C. Roger Bannister

D. Sebastian Coe

49. *Which team won the NBA Championship in 1950?*

A — Boston Celtics

B — Minneapolis Lakers

C — Philadelphia Warriors

D — New York Knicks

50. *The 'Miracle Mile' featured a race between which two runners?*

A — Emil Z?topek and Alain Mimoun

B — Roger Bannister and John Landy

C — Paavo Nurmi and Jim Ryun

D — Sebastian Coe and Steve Ovett

51. *Which country won the most medals in the 1952 Helsinki Olympics?*

A — United States

B — Soviet Union

C — Finland

D — Sweden

52. *Who was the first driver to win the Indianapolis 500 three times?*

A — A.J. Foyt

B — Al Unser

C — Mauri Rose

D — Wilbur Shaw

53. *Which woman won Wimbledon in 1957 after having a baby?*

A. Maureen Connolly

B. Althea Gibson

C. Doris Hart

D. Shirley Fry

54. *What was the nickname of the 1950s Hungarian national football team?*

A. The Red Devils

B. The Magical Magyars

C. The Azzurri

D. The Oranje

55. *Which horse won the Triple Crown in 1956?*

A. Citation

B. Assault

C. Count Fleet

D. Needles

56. *Which athlete set a world record in the long jump at the 1956 Olympics?*

A. Bob Beamon

B. Jesse Owens

C. Greg Louganis

D. Bob Mathias

57. *Who was the first African American to play in the NBA?*

A. Bill Russell

B. Wilt Chamberlain

C. Earl Lloyd

D. Elgin Baylor

58. *Which team won the NHL Stanley Cup in 1950?*

A. Toronto Maple Leafs

B. Montreal Canadiens

C. Detroit Red Wings

D. New York Rangers

59. *What major event in auto racing began in 1950?*

A. Daytona 500

B. Formula One World Championship

C. Indianapolis 500

D. Le Mans 24 Hours

60. *Who won the Tour de France in 1950?*

A. Gino Bartali

B. Jacques Anquetil

C. Fausto Coppi

D. Louison Bobet

61. *Which state became the 50th of the United States in 1959?*

A. Alaska
B. Hawaii
C. Puerto Rico
D. Guam

62. *Who became the Prime Minister of the United Kingdom in 1955?*

A. Winston Churchill
B. Harold Macmillan
C. Anthony Eden
D. Clement Attlee

63. *The Korean War ended in which year?*

A. 1950
B. 1953
C. 1955
D. 1957

64. *What was launched into space during the International Geophysical Year?*

A. Hubble Telescope
B. Sputnik 1
C. Explorer 1
D. Voyager 1

65. *Which landmark U.S. Supreme Court case declared school segregation unconstitutional?*

A. Plessy v. Ferguson

B. Brown v. Board of Education

C. Roe v. Wade

D. Miranda v. Arizona

66. *Which leader started the 'Great Leap Forward' in 1958?*

A. Mao Zedong

B. Nikita Khrushchev

C. Ho Chi Minh

D. Kim Il-sung

67. *What was the first commercial jet airliner to enter service in 1952?*

A. Boeing 707

B. Douglas DC-8

C. De Havilland Comet

D. Lockheed Constellation

68. *The 'Battle of Dien Bien Phu' was a pivotal moment in which conflict?*

A. Korean War

B. Vietnam War

C. Suez Crisis

D. Algerian War

69. *Which country gained independence from Britain in 1957, becoming the first African country to do so?*

A) Nigeria	B) Kenya
C) Ghana	D) South Africa

70. *The Treaty of Rome, creating the European Economic Community, was signed in what year?*

A) 1950	B) 1957
C) 1960	D) 1963

71. *Which iconic structure in France was completed in 1958?*

A) The Louvre Pyramid	B) Centre Pompidou
C) Montparnasse Tower	D) UNESCO Headquarters

72. *Who led the Cuban Revolution in 1959?*

A) Fulgencio Batista	B) Che Guevara
C) Fidel Castro	D) Ra?l Castro

73. *The Antarctic Treaty was signed in which year?*

A	1950	B	1959
C	1961	D	1967

74. *What was the name of the first nuclear-powered submarine launched in 1954?*

A	USS Nautilus	B	USS Enterprise
C	USS Nimitz	D	USS Triton

75. *Which event marked the beginning of the Space Race?*

A	The Apollo Program	B	The launch of Sputnik 1
C	The founding of NASA	D	The Moon landing

76. *Which conference led to the creation of the Warsaw Pact in 1955?*

A	Yalta Conference	B	Potsdam Conference
C	Geneva Conference	D	Paris Peace Treaties

77. *Who was the American Vice President under Dwight D. Eisenhower?*

A	Harry S. Truman	B	Lyndon B. Johnson
C	Richard Nixon	D	John F. Kennedy

78. *The first 'Miss Universe' pageant was held in which year?*

A	1950	B	1952
C	1955	D	1958

79. *Which country launched the first satellite, Sputnik, into space?*

A	United States	B	Soviet Union
C	United Kingdom	D	France

80. *What was the name of the first artificial Earth satellite?*

A	Explorer 1	B	Vanguard 1
C	Telstar	D	Sputnik 1

81. *What was the first successful vaccine developed in the 1950s?*

A. Polio Vaccine

B. Measles Vaccine

C. Mumps Vaccine

D. Rubella Vaccine

82. *Who invented the first commercially successful transistor radio?*

A. Sony

B. Motorola

C. RCA

D. Philips

83. *Which scientist discovered the structure of DNA in 1953?*

A. Rosalind Franklin

B. James Watson and Francis Crick

C. Linus Pauling

D. Maurice Wilkins

84. *The first practical solar cell was demonstrated in which year?*

A. 1954

B. 1951

C. 1957

D. 1959

85. *'Velcro' was invented by George de Mestral after being inspired by what?*

A	Sea Urchins	B	Honeycomb
C	Bird Feathers	D	Burdock Burrs

86. *Which computer language was developed by IBM in the 1950s?*

A	COBOL	B	FORTRAN
C	BASIC	D	Assembly

87. *The first artificial heart was invented by whom?*

A	Willem Kolff	B	Christiaan Barnard
C	Michael DeBakey	D	Robert Jarvik

88. *What was the first video game created in 1958?*

A	Pong	B	Spacewar!
C	Tennis for Two	D	Asteroids

89. *Who is credited with inventing the microchip?*

A) Gordon Moore	B) Jack Kilby
C) Robert Noyce	D) William Shockley

90. *The first satellite to be solar-powered was launched in which year?*

A) 1957	B) 1958
C) 1959	D) 1960

91. *Which antibiotic was first used in the 1950s to treat tuberculosis?*

A) Penicillin	B) Streptomycin
C) Tetracycline	D) Erythromycin

92. *The first successful weather satellite was launched in which year?*

A) 1952	B) 1954
C) 1957	D) 1960

93. *Who developed the first effective polio vaccine?*

A) Albert Sabin
B) Jonas Salk
C) Louis Pasteur
D) Alexander Fleming

94. *What was the first animal to orbit the Earth?*

A) A monkey
B) A dog
C) A mouse
D) A cat

95. *The discovery of which element's isotopes led to the development of the atomic clock?*

A) Uranium
B) Cesium
C) Hydrogen
D) Carbon

96. *Which space probe was the first to photograph the far side of the Moon?*

A) Luna 1
B) Luna 2
C) Luna 3
D) Mariner 2

97. *The first organ transplant was performed in which year?*

A	1950	B	1954
C	1958	D	1962

98. *Who was awarded the Nobel Prize in Physics for the invention of the transistor?*

A	Enrico Fermi	B	Niels Bohr
C	William Shockley	D	Werner Heisenberg

99. *What innovation in timekeeping was introduced in 1955?*

A	Digital Watch	B	Quartz Clock
C	Atomic Clock	D	Solar-Powered Watch

100. *'Myxomatosis' was introduced to control the rabbit population in which country?*

A	United States	B	United Kingdom
C	Australia	D	New Zealand

The 1960's

The Swinging 1960s: A Decade of Revolution and Expression

The 1960s were a seismic shift of culture and consciousness. It was a decade marked by the rise of civil rights, the fervor of anti-war protests, and the sound of The Beatles echoing across the Atlantic. This was a time when the world witnessed profound social changes, space exploration reached new heights, and the youth challenged the status quo.

From the miniskirts to the moon landing, the '60s redefined freedom and set the stage for innovation. It was an era where television brought global events into living rooms, music festivals became symbols of peace, and movements for equality gained momentum.

As you delve into the trivia of the 1960s, get ready to relive the passion of Woodstock, the speeches of Martin Luther King Jr., and the race to space that captured the imagination of millions. The 1960s were not just years; they were the canvas of modern history.

Let's test your knowledge of this revolutionary decade!

101. *Who released the hit song "I Can't Get No Satisfaction" in 1965?*

A. The Beatles
B. The Beach Boys
C. The Rolling Stones
D. The Kinks

102. *Which music festival of 1969 is remembered for its iconic performances and cultural impact?*

A. Monterey Pop Festival
B. Woodstock
C. Isle of Wight Festival
D. Altamont Free Concert

103. *Who was the famous female soul singer known for "Respect" in 1967?*

A. Diana Ross
B. Aretha Franklin
C. Tina Turner
D. Janis Joplin

104. *What was the name of the dance craze popularized by Chubby Checker in the 1960s?*

A. The Twist
B. The Mashed Potato
C. The Loco-Motion
D. The Shimmy

105. *Which band's album "Sgt. Pepper's Lonely Hearts Club Band" was a huge hit in 1967?*

A. The Who

B. Pink Floyd

C. The Beatles

D. The Rolling Stones

106. *Which song by The Doors became a hit in 1967?*

A. Light My Fire

B. Riders on the Storm

C. Break On Through

D. The End

107. *Who was the lead singer of The Supremes in the 1960s?*

A. Martha Reeves

B. Diana Ross

C. Mary Wells

D. Tammi Terrell

108. *What was the title of the 1968 hit by Simon & Garfunkel?*

A. Bridge Over Troubled Water

B. The Sound of Silence

C. Mrs. Robinson

D. Cecilia

109. *Which band is known for the song "California Dreamin'" released in 1965?*

A. The Mamas & the Papas
B. The Byrds
C. The Beach Boys
D. Buffalo Springfield

110. *"Born to Be Wild" was a 1968 hit for which rock band?*

A. Steppenwolf
B. The Animals
C. Jefferson Airplane
D. The Yardbirds

111. *Which artist is known for the song "Blowin' in the Wind" released in 1963?*

A. Bob Dylan
B. Neil Young
C. Joni Mitchell
D. Jimi Hendrix

112. *The Beatles' album "Revolver" was released in which year?*

A. 1965
B. 1966
C. 1967
D. 1968

113. *Who performed the hit "My Girl" in 1964?*

A	The Temptations	B	The Four Tops
C	The Drifters	D	The Platters

114. *What is the name of the iconic guitar riff in "Satisfaction" by The Rolling Stones?*

A	The Last Time	B	Jumpin' Jack Flash
C	Paint It Black	D	Keith's Riff

115. *"Space Oddity," a song about an astronaut, was released by which artist?*

A	David Bowie	B	Elton John
C	Lou Reed	D	Leonard Cohen

116. *Which band had a hit with "A Whiter Shade of Pale" in 1967?*

A	The Moody Blues	B	Procol Harum
C	The Zombies	D	Cream

117. *"The Sound of Silence" is a classic hit by which duo?*

A. Sonny & Cher

B. Simon & Garfunkel

C. Jan & Dean

D. Ike & Tina Turner

118. *What was Jimi Hendrix's famous closing performance at Woodstock '69?*

A. Purple Haze

B. Foxy Lady

C. The Star-Spangled Banner

D. Voodoo Child

119. *Which song by The Beatles begins with the lyrics "Picture yourself in a boat on a river"?*

A. Yellow Submarine

B. Eleanor Rigby

C. Lucy in the Sky with Diamonds

D. Let It Be

120. *Who is known for the 1961 hit "Stand By Me"?*

A. Marvin Gaye

B. Otis Redding

C. Ben E. King

D. Sam Cooke

121. *Which film won the Academy Award for Best Picture in 1960?*

A. Spartacus

B. Psycho

C. The Apartment

D. Exodus

122. *Who starred as the title character in the 1960s TV series "Batman"?*

A. Adam West

B. Burt Ward

C. Michael Keaton

D. George Clooney

123. *What 1964 film featured the song "Supercalifragilisticexpialidocious"?*

A. The Sound of Music

B. Mary Poppins

C. My Fair Lady

D. Chitty Chitty Bang Bang

124. *Which actor played the role of Norman Bates in "Psycho" (1960)?*

A. Anthony Perkins

B. Jack Nicholson

C. Tony Curtis

D. Gregory Peck

125. *The TV show "Star Trek" debuted in which year?*

A. 1963
B. 1966
C. 1969
D. 1960

126. *Who directed the epic historical drama "Lawrence of Arabia" released in 1962?*

A. Alfred Hitchcock
B. Stanley Kubrick
C. David Lean
D. John Ford

127. *Which actress starred as Eliza Doolittle in "My Fair Lady" (1964)?*

A. Julie Andrews
B. Audrey Hepburn
C. Elizabeth Taylor
D. Sophia Loren

128. *The classic TV show "The Twilight Zone" ended in which year?*

A. 1960
B. 1962
C. 1964
D. 1967

129. *What was the first James Bond film released in the 1960s?*

A Goldfinger	**B** Dr. No
C From Russia with Love	**D** Thunderball

130. *"The Pink Panther" series featured which actor as Inspector Clouseau?*

A Sean Connery	**B** Peter Sellers
C Steve McQueen	**D** Richard Burton

131. *Which 1960 film is famous for its shower scene?*

A Vertigo	**B** Psycho
C The Birds	**D** North by Northwest

132. *Who hosted the popular game show "The Price Is Right" when it debuted in 1965?*

A Bob Barker	**B** Bill Cullen
C Garry Moore	**D** Jack Barry

133. *"The Man from U.N.C.L.E." was a spy-fi TV series that aired starting in which year?*

A 1960	B 1962
C 1964	D 1966

134. *What is the name of the spaceship in the 1960s TV series "Lost in Space"?*

A Enterprise	B Jupiter 2
C Millennium Falcon	D Galactica

135. *Which actress played the role of Catwoman in the 1960s "Batman" TV series?*

A Julie Newmar	B Eartha Kitt
C Lee Meriwether	D Michelle Pfeiffer

136. *Which movie features the character Atticus Finch, a lawyer in a racially charged trial?*

A To Kill a Mockingbird	B In the Heat of the Night
C Guess Who's Coming to Dinner	D The Defiant Ones

137. *"Gilligan's Island" is a TV show about castaways on an uncharted island. When did it first air?*

A	1960	B	1962
C	1964	D	1967

138. *Who played the lead role in the 1963 film "Cleopatra"?*

A	Vivien Leigh	B	Elizabeth Taylor
C	Sophia Loren	D	Audrey Hepburn

139. *What was the name of the spy portrayed by Michael Caine in the "Harry Palmer" series?*

A	James Bond	B	Ethan Hunt
C	Harry Palmer	D	Jason Bourne

140. *Which 1960s TV show's theme song had the lyrics "They're creepy and they're kooky, mysterious and spooky"?*

A	The Twilight Zone	B	The Munsters
C	The Addams Family	D	Bewitched

141. *Who set the men's long jump world record at the 1968 Olympics?*

A Carl Lewis	B Jesse Owens
C Bob Beamon	D Mike Powell

142. *Which country hosted the 1964 Summer Olympics?*

A Mexico	B Japan
C Italy	D United States

143. *What was Muhammad Ali's original name before changing it in 1964?*

A Cassius Clay	B Malcolm X
C Lew Alcindor	D Jim Brown

144. *Which football team won the first Super Bowl in 1967?*

A Green Bay Packers	B Kansas City Chiefs
C New York Jets	D Dallas Cowboys

145. *Who won the Tour de France five consecutive times starting in 1961?*

A. Eddy Merckx

B. Jacques Anquetil

C. Bernard Hinault

D. Miguel Indurain

146. *Which famous golfer won the Masters Tournament four times during the 1960s?*

A. Gary Player

B. Jack Nicklaus

C. Arnold Palmer

D. Lee Trevino

147. *What significant event in the history of baseball occurred in 1961?*

A. The first World Series night game

B. The first use of instant replay

C. Roger Maris broke Babe Ruth's home run record

D. The first baseball game broadcast in color

148. *Who was the heavyweight boxing champion at the end of the 1960s?*

A. Floyd Patterson

B. Joe Frazier

C. Muhammad Ali

D. George Foreman

149. *Which country won the FIFA World Cup in 1966?*

A. Brazil

B. Italy

C. England

D. West Germany

150. *In 1967, Kathrine Switzer became the first woman to do what?*

A. Win an Olympic gold medal

B. Run the Boston Marathon as a numbered entry

C. Swim the English Channel

D. Compete in the Indy 500

151. *Which athlete was named "Sportsman of the Century" by Sports Illustrated in 1960?*

A. Muhammad Ali

B. Jim Brown

C. Bill Russell

D. Rafer Johnson

152. *Who won the first official NASCAR Grand National Championship in 1960?*

A. Richard Petty

B. Lee Petty

C. Junior Johnson

D. David Pearson

153. *Which NHL team won five Stanley Cup titles in the 1960s?*

A. Toronto Maple Leafs

B. Montreal Canadiens

C. Detroit Red Wings

D. Boston Bruins

154. *What was the original name of the AFL team known as the Kansas City Chiefs in the 1960s?*

A. Dallas Texans

B. Houston Oilers

C. Buffalo Bills

D. Denver Broncos

155. *In 1960, which country became the first to win three European Football Championships?*

A. Italy

B. West Germany

C. Soviet Union

D. Spain

156. *Which famous horse won the Triple Crown in 1966?*

A. Secretariat

B. Seattle Slew

C. Affirmed

D. Sir Barton

157. *Who was the first gymnast to score a perfect 10.0 in the Olympics?*

A	Olga Korbut	B	Nadia Com?neci
C	Larisa Latynina	D	Mary Lou Retton

158. *Which team won the first ever Super Bowl in 1967?*

A	Green Bay Packers	B	Kansas City Chiefs
C	New York Jets	D	Dallas Cowboys

159. *Who was the dominant female tennis player of the 1960s, winning 19 Grand Slam titles?*

A	Billie Jean King	B	Margaret Court
C	Maria Bueno	D	Chris Evert

160. *What was the significant achievement of Wilt Chamberlain in the NBA in 1962?*

A	Winning the MVP Award	B	Scoring 100 points in a single game
C	Highest season scoring average	D	Winning the NBA Championship

161. *Which event marked the beginning of the space race in 1961?*

A) Apollo 11 Moon Landing

B) Yuri Gagarin's Orbit

C) Gemini Program Launch

D) Sputnik Satellite Launch

162. *Who became the first female Prime Minister of a country in 1960?*

A) Golda Meir

B) Indira Gandhi

C) Margaret Thatcher

D) Sirimavo Bandaranaike

163. *The Berlin Wall was constructed in which year?*

A) 1961

B) 1962

C) 1963

D) 1964

164. *What was the main goal of the Civil Rights Act, signed into law in 1964?*

A) Women's Suffrage

B) Prohibition of Alcohol

C) Ending Racial Segregation

D) Voting Rights for 18-Year-Olds

165. *The Cuban Missile Crisis occurred in which year?*

A. 1960
B. 1961
C. 1962
D. 1963

166. *Which U.S. President signed the Civil Rights Act into law in 1964?*

A. John F. Kennedy
B. Lyndon B. Johnson
C. Richard Nixon
D. Dwight D. Eisenhower

167. *The "Summer of Love" primarily took place in which city in 1967?*

A. New York
B. San Francisco
C. Los Angeles
D. Chicago

168. *What was the name of the American pilot shot down over the Soviet Union in 1960?*

A. John Glenn
B. Alan Shepard
C. Gary Powers
D. Chuck Yeager

169. *Who was the influential leader of the Soviet Union during most of the 1960s?*

A) Leonid Brezhnev

B) Nikita Khrushchev

C) Joseph Stalin

D) Mikhail Gorbachev

170. *The landmark U.S. Supreme Court case "Miranda v. Arizona" established what?*

A) The right to free speech

B) The right to bear arms

C) The right to an attorney

D) The right to privacy

171. *Which U.S. President established the Peace Corps in 1961?*

A) John F. Kennedy

B) Lyndon B. Johnson

C) Richard Nixon

D) Dwight D. Eisenhower

172. *The Six-Day War in 1967 was fought between Israel and which countries?*

A) Egypt, Jordan, and Syria

B) Iraq, Iran, and Turkey

C) Lebanon, Saudi Arabia, and Yemen

D) Kuwait, Algeria, and Libya

173. *What was the major environmental disaster that struck the UK in 1967?*

A The Great Smog

B The Torrey Canyon oil spill

C The Aberfan disaster

D The North Sea flood

174. *Who assassinated U.S. presidential candidate Robert F. Kennedy in 1968?*

A Lee Harvey Oswald

B James Earl Ray

C Sirhan Sirhan

D Jack Ruby

175. *Which amendment to the U.S. Constitution, ratified in 1964, abolished poll taxes?*

A 22nd Amendment

B 23rd Amendment

C 24th Amendment

D 25th Amendment

176. *Which spacecraft completed the first manned orbit of the Moon in 1968?*

A Apollo 7

B Apollo 8

C Apollo 9

D Apollo 10

177. *Who was the first woman to travel into space, doing so in 1963?*

A. Sally Ride

B. Valentina Tereshkova

C. Mae Jemison

D. Eileen Collins

178. *The Voting Rights Act, prohibiting racial discrimination in voting, was enacted in what year?*

A. 1962

B. 1964

C. 1965

D. 1967

179. *Which U.S. President declared the "War on Poverty" in 1964?*

A. John F. Kennedy

B. Lyndon B. Johnson

C. Richard Nixon

D. Dwight D. Eisenhower

180. *What was the pivotal event of the Vietnam War that began on January 30, 1968?*

A. The Gulf of Tonkin Incident

B. The Tet Offensive

C. The Battle of Khe Sanh

D. The My Lai Massacre

181. *Which invention by Douglas Engelbart revolutionized computer input devices in 1968?*

A. The Keyboard

B. The Mouse

C. The Monitor

D. The Printer

182. *The first successful heart transplant was performed by Dr. Christiaan Barnard in which year?*

A. 1967

B. 1968

C. 1969

D. 1966

183. *What was the name of the first video game, simulating table tennis, released in 1966?*

A. Pong

B. Spacewar!

C. Asteroids

D. Pac-Man

184. *Who developed the first laser in 1960?*

A. Gordon Gould

B. Theodore Maiman

C. Charles Townes

D. Arthur Schawlow

185. *"Silent Spring," a book that led to a ban on DDT, was published by Rachel Carson in what year?*

A	1960	B	1961
C	1962	D	1963

186. *What significant medical device was invented by Wilson Greatbatch in 1960?*

A	The Pacemaker	B	The MRI Machine
C	The Ultrasound	D	The Dialysis Machine

187. *Which space mission first landed humans on the Moon in 1969?*

A	Apollo 10	B	Apollo 11
C	Apollo 12	D	Apollo 13

188. *The first communication satellite, Telstar, was launched in what year?*

A	1960	B	1962
C	1964	D	1966

189. *Kevlar, a high-strength material, was invented by Stephanie Kwolek in which year?*

A. 1965

B. 1967

C. 1971

D. 1975

190. *Who was awarded the Nobel Prize in Physics in 1965 for his work on quantum electrodynamics? *

A. Niels Bohr

B. Werner Heisenberg

C. Richard Feynman

D. Paul Dirac

191. *Who invented the first practical optical fiber for telecommunications in 1966?*

A. Charles K. Kao

B. John Logie Baird

C. Alexander Graham Bell

D. Guglielmo Marconi

192. *The first handheld calculator was introduced by which company in 1967?*

A. IBM

B. Texas Instruments

C. Casio

D. Hewlett-Packard

193. *Which space probe performed the first flyby of Mars in 1965?*

A. Voyager 1

B. Sputnik

C. Mariner 4

D. Pioneer 10

194. *The discovery of the cosmic microwave background radiation in 1965 supported which theory?*

A. Steady State Theory

B. Big Bang Theory

C. Plasma Cosmology

D. Pulsating Universe Theory

195. *What was the name of the first weather satellite launched by NASA in 1960?*

A. GOES

B. Meteosat

C. TIROS-1

D. Landsat

196. *Which Apollo mission was the first to successfully dock with another spacecraft in orbit?*

A. Apollo 7

B. Apollo 9

C. Apollo 10

D. Apollo 11

197. *Who developed the polio vaccine announced as safe in 1960?*

A. Albert Sabin
B. Jonas Salk
C. Louis Pasteur
D. Alexander Fleming

198. *The first geostationary communications satellite, Syncom, was launched in which year?*

A. 1961
B. 1963
C. 1965
D. 1967

199. *What was the name of the first quasar discovered in 1963?*

A. PKS 1004+13
B. 3C 273
C. M87
D. Cygnus A

200. *The first demonstration of ARPANET, the precursor to the internet, was in what year?*

A. 1967
B. 1969
C. 1971
D. 1973

The 1970's

The Dynamic 1970s: A Decade of Disco, Diversity, and Discovery

The 1970s were a colorful tapestry of change, a time when the disco ball spun over a generation exploring new freedoms. It was an era that danced to the beat of its own drum, from the glitter of Studio 54 to the groundbreaking strides in civil rights and environmental awareness.

This decade saw the end of the Vietnam War, the Watergate scandal, and the rise of personal computing. It was a time when music went from the earthy tones of folk to the electronic pulse of disco, and fashion made its own rules with bell-bottoms and platform shoes.

As you turn the pages to the trivia of the 1970s, get ready to revisit the era of 'Star Wars', the fervor of the feminist movement, and the first steps of the technological revolution that would shape the future. The 1970s were bold, brash, and unapologetically brilliant.

Let's rediscover the spirit of this transformative decade!

201. *Which band released the album "Dark Side of the Moon" in 1973?*

A Pink Floyd

B Led Zeppelin

C The Beatles

D The Rolling Stones

202. *Which singer-songwriter won the Nobel Prize in Literature in 2016 for his lyrics?*

A Bob Dylan

B John Lennon

C Paul Simon

D Leonard Cohen

203. *Which disco group had a hit with the song "Stayin' Alive" in 1977?*

A ABBA

B Bee Gees

C Village People

D Earth, Wind & Fire

204. *Which rock opera by The Who was adapted into a film in 1975?*

A Tommy

B Quadrophenia

C Jesus Christ Superstar

D Hair

205. *Which musical genre emerged in the late 1970s as a reaction to mainstream rock?*

A. Punk

B. Reggae

C. Funk

D. Soul

206. *Which Swedish pop group won the Eurovision Song Contest in 1974 with the song "Waterloo"?*

A. ABBA

B. Roxette

C. Ace of Base

D. A-ha

207. *Which rock band featured siblings Ann and Nancy Wilson as lead singers?*

A. Heart

B. Fleetwood Mac

C. The Bangles

D. The Carpenters

208. *Which singer was known as the "King of Rock and Roll" until his death in 1977?*

A. Elvis Presley

B. Chuck Berry

C. Little Richard

D. Jerry Lee Lewis

209. *Which song by Queen became a hit again in 1992 after being featured in the movie "Wayne's World"?*

A	We Will Rock You	B	Another One Bites the Dust
C	Bohemian Rhapsody	D	We Are the Champions

210. *Which musical instrument did Stevie Wonder play despite being blind?*

A	Piano	B	Guitar
C	Violin	D	Saxophone

211. *Which British rock band had a hit with the song "Stairway to Heaven" in 1971?*

A	The Beatles	B	The Rolling Stones
C	Led Zeppelin	D	The Who

212. *Which American singer was nicknamed the "Boss" and released the album "Born to Run" in 1975?*

A	Bruce Springsteen	B	Bob Seger
C	Tom Petty	D	John Mellencamp

213. *Which Jamaican singer popularized reggae music in the 1970s with songs like "No Woman, No Cry" and "One Love"?*

A. Bob Marley

B. Jimmy Cliff

C. Peter Tosh

D. Desmond Dekker

214. *Which musical film starring John Travolta and Olivia Newton-John was released in 1978 and became a global phenomenon?*

A. Saturday Night Fever

B. Grease

C. Dirty Dancing

D. Footloose

215. *Which Australian rock band had a hit with the song "Highway to Hell" in 1979?*

A. AC/DC

B. INXS

C. Men at Work

D. Midnight Oil

216. *Which American singer-songwriter released the album "Tapestry" in 1971, which became one of the best-selling albums of all time?*

A. Carole King

B. Joni Mitchell

C. Carly Simon

D. Janis Joplin

217. *Which British rock band had a hit with the song "Bohemian Rhapsody" in 1975, which featured an operatic section?*

A) Queen
B) The Beatles
C) The Rolling Stones
D) The Who

218. *Which American funk band had a hit with the song "Le Freak" in 1978, which was inspired by being denied entry to Studio 54?*

A) Earth, Wind & Fire
B) Kool & the Gang
C) Chic
D) The Commodores

219. *Which musical film starring John Travolta and Olivia Newton-John was released in 1978 and became a global phenomenon?*

A) Saturday Night Fever
B) Grease
C) Dirty Dancing
D) Footloose

220. *Which American singer was known as the "Queen of Disco" and had hits with songs like "I Feel Love" and "Last Dance"?*

A) Donna Summer
B) Gloria Gaynor
C) Diana Ross
D) Tina Turner

221. *Which movie won the Academy Award for Best Picture in 1972?*

A. The Godfather

B. The French Connection

C. Cabaret

D. Deliverance

222. *Which TV show featured a family of seven children living in a rural Virginia town during the Great Depression and World War II?*

A. Little House on the Prairie

B. The Waltons

C. The Brady Bunch

D. Happy Days

223. *Which actor played the role of Rocky Balboa, a struggling boxer who gets a chance to fight the heavyweight champion, in the 1976 movie Rocky?*

A. Sylvester Stallone

B. Robert De Niro

C. Al Pacino

D. Clint Eastwood

224. *Which TV show featured a group of women working at a fictional radio station in Cincinnati, Ohio?*

A. The Mary Tyler Moore Show

B. Laverne & Shirley

C. WKRP in Cincinnati

D. Charlie's Angels

225. *Which movie was based on the novel by Stephen King and featured a teenage girl with telekinetic powers?*

A	The Exorcist	B	The Omen
C	Carrie	D	The Shining

226. *Which movie starred Jack Nicholson as a writer who goes insane while staying at a haunted hotel?*

A	The Shining	B	The Exorcist
C	Psycho	D	The Amityville Horror

227. *Which TV show featured a family of four who lived in a futuristic apartment with a robot maid named Rosie?*

A	The Jetsons	B	The Flintstones
C	Lost in Space	D	Star Trek

228. *Which movie was based on the true story of a group of prisoners who escaped from a German POW camp during World War II?*

A	The Great Escape	B	The Bridge on the River Kwai
C	The Dirty Dozen	D	The Guns of Navarone

229. *Which TV show featured a detective who solved crimes using his "little grey cells" and his trademark moustache?*

A Columbo

B Sherlock Holmes

C Poirot

D Magnum, P.I.

230. *Which movie starred John Wayne as a veteran of the Vietnam War who returns to his hometown and faces hostility from the locals?*

A The Green Berets

B The Deer Hunter

C The Searchers

D The Quiet Man

231. *Which movie starred Dustin Hoffman as a college graduate who has an affair with an older woman?*

A The Graduate

B Midnight Cowboy

C Kramer vs. Kramer

D Tootsie

232. *Which TV show featured a team of undercover cops who used unconventional methods to fight crime?*

A Starsky & Hutch

B Hawaii Five-O

C The A-Team

D Miami Vice

233. *Which movie was based on the novel by Mario Puzo and featured Marlon Brando as the head of a powerful mafia family?*

A The Godfather	**B** Goodfellas
C Scarface	**D** The Untouchables

234. *Which TV show featured a group of friends who lived in a New York apartment building and often hung out at a coffee shop?*

A Friends	**B** Seinfeld
C Cheers	**D** The Odd Couple

235. *Which movie starred Gene Wilder as a candy maker who invites five children to tour his factory? *

A Willy Wonka & the Chocolate Factory	**B** Charlie and the Chocolate Factory
C Chitty Chitty Bang Bang	**D** Mary Poppins

236. *Which movie starred Robert Redford and Paul Newman as two con artists who pull off a complicated scam?*

A The Sting	**B** Butch Cassidy and the Sundance Kid
C The Hustler	**D** The Great Gatsby

237. *Which TV show featured a wealthy oil tycoon and his family who lived in a mansion in Dallas, Texas?*

A. Dynasty

B. Dallas

C. Falcon Crest

D. Knots Landing

238. *Which movie starred Woody Allen as a neurotic comedian who falls in love with an aspiring singer played by Diane Keaton?*

A. Annie Hall

B. Manhattan

C. Hannah and Her Sisters

D. Sleeper

239. *Which TV show featured a young woman who worked as a private investigator for her father's agency?*

A. Charlie's Angels

B. The Bionic Woman

C. Wonder Woman

D. Nancy Drew

240. *Which movie starred Clint Eastwood as a rogue cop who uttered the famous line "Go ahead, make my day"?*

A. Dirty Harry

B. Magnum Force

C. Sudden Impact

D. The Enforcer

241. *Which country won the FIFA World Cup in 1970, becoming the first team to win three titles?*

A Brazil	B Italy
C Germany	D Argentina

242. *Which tennis player won the Wimbledon men's singles title seven times in the 1970s?*

A Bjorn Borg	B John McEnroe
C Jimmy Connors	D Rod Laver

243. *Which Formula One driver won his first world championship in 1975 and survived a near-fatal crash in 1976?*

A Jackie Stewart	B Niki Lauda
C James Hunt	D Emerson Fittipaldi

244. *Which sport was introduced to the Olympic Games for the first time in 1972?*

A Badminton	B Handball
C Taekwondo	D Table tennis

245. *Which boxer defeated Muhammad Ali in 1971 in what was dubbed as "The Fight of the Century"?*

A	Joe Frazier	B	George Foreman
C	Ken Norton	D	Sonny Liston

246. *Which basketball player led the Boston Celtics to six NBA championships in the 1970s?*

A	Larry Bird	B	Bill Russell
C	Kareem Abdul-Jabbar	D	John Havlicek

247. *Which sportswear company was founded in 1971 by Phil Knight and Bill Bowerman?*

A	Adidas	B	Nike
C	Reebok	D	Puma

248. *Which Olympic gymnast scored a perfect 10 for the first time in history in 1976?*

A	Olga Korbut	B	Nadia Comaneci
C	Mary Lou Retton	D	Larisa Latynina

249. *Which soccer player scored the winning goal for West Germany in the 1974 World Cup final against the Netherlands?*

A) Franz Beckenbauer

B) Gerd Muller

C) Uwe Seeler

D) Karl-Heinz Rummenigge

250. *Which golf legend won his record 18th major championship in 1978?*

A) Jack Nicklaus

B) Arnold Palmer

C) Gary Player

D) Tom Watson

251. *Which American swimmer won seven gold medals at the 1972 Munich Olympics, setting a new record?*

A) Mark Spitz

B) Michael Phelps

C) Johnny Weissmuller

D) Matt Biondi

252. *Which British athlete broke the four-minute mile barrier for the first time in 1975?*

A) Roger Bannister

B) Sebastian Coe

C) Steve Ovett

D) John Walker

253. *Which sport was banned in China from 1966 to 1976 as part of the Cultural Revolution?*

A. Soccer

B. Basketball

C. Ping pong

D. Chess

254. *Which American football team won four Super Bowls in the 1970s?*

A. Dallas Cowboys

B. Pittsburgh Steelers

C. San Francisco 49ers

D. Miami Dolphins

255. *Which Canadian ice hockey player scored his first NHL goal in 1979 and went on to become the all-time leading scorer in the league?*

A. Wayne Gretzky

B. Mario Lemieux

C. Bobby Orr

D. Gordie Howe

256. *Which British cyclist won the Tour de France in 1978, becoming the first and only rider from his country to do so?*

A. Bradley Wiggins

B. Chris Froome

C. Tom Simpson

D. Bernard Hinault

257. *Which sport was dominated by the Soviet Union in the 1970s, winning six consecutive Olympic gold medals?*

A. Basketball

B. Hockey

C. Volleyball

D. Wrestling

258. *Which American baseball player broke Babe Ruth's career home run record in 1974?*

A. Hank Aaron

B. Willie Mays

C. Mickey Mantle

D. Reggie Jackson

259. *Which martial arts legend starred in the 1973 movie Enter the Dragon, which was released after his death?*

A. Bruce Lee

B. Jackie Chan

C. Jet Li

D. Chuck Norris

260. *Which sport was banned in South Africa from 1970 to 1991 due to the apartheid policy?*

A. Rugby

B. Cricket

C. Soccer

D. Golf

261. *Which U.S. president resigned from office in 1974 after the Watergate scandal?*

A. Richard Nixon
B. Gerald Ford
C. Jimmy Carter
D. Ronald Reagan

262. *Which Asian country was divided into two states after the end of the Vietnam War in 1975?*

A. Korea
B. China
C. Vietnam
D. Cambodia

263. *Which Middle Eastern country was invaded by the Soviet Union in 1979, sparking a decade-long war?*

A. Iran
B. Iraq
C. Afghanistan
D. Pakistan

264. *Which revolutionary leader overthrew the monarchy of Iran in 1979 and established an Islamic republic?*

A. Saddam Hussein
B. Yasser Arafat
C. Muammar Gaddafi
D. Ruhollah Khomeini

265. *Which African country gained its independence from Portugal in 1975 after a long guerrilla war?*

A. Angola
B. Mozambique
C. Zimbabwe
D. South Africa

266. *Which European country was ruled by a military dictatorship until 1974, when a peaceful revolution restored democracy?*

A. Spain
B. Portugal
C. Greece
D. Italy

267. *Which terrorist group kidnapped and killed 11 Israeli athletes at the 1972 Munich Olympics?*

A. Al-Qaeda
B. IRA
C. ETA
D. Black September

268. *Which landmark agreement was signed in 1978 by the leaders of Egypt and Israel, ending decades of conflict?*

A. Camp David Accords
B. Oslo Accords
C. Geneva Convention
D. Treaty of Versailles

269. *Which Southeast Asian country was devastated by the genocide of the Khmer Rouge regime from 1975 to 1979?*

A. Vietnam

B. Laos

C. Cambodia

D. Thailand

270. *Which Chinese leader initiated the economic reforms and the opening up of China to the world in 1978?*

A. Mao Zedong

B. Deng Xiaoping

C. Zhou Enlai

D. Chiang Kai-shek

271. *Which South American country was ruled by a brutal military dictatorship from 1976 to 1983, known as the "Dirty War"?*

A. Chile

B. Argentina

C. Brazil

D. Colombia

272. *Which British prime minister was elected in 1979, becoming the first woman to hold the position?*

A. Margaret Thatcher

B. Theresa May

C. Indira Gandhi

D. Angela Merkel

273. *Which space station was launched by the Soviet Union in 1971 and remained in orbit until 2001?*

A. Salyut

B. Skylab

C. Mir

D. ISS

274. *Which civil rights activist and Nobel Peace Prize winner was assassinated in 1978 in San Francisco?*

A. Martin Luther King Jr.

B. Malcolm X

C. Harvey Milk

D. Nelson Mandela

275. *Which Southeast Asian country was invaded by Vietnam in 1978, ending the rule of the Khmer Rouge?*

A. Laos

B. Thailand

C. Cambodia

D. Myanmar

276. *Which anti-apartheid activist and Nobel Peace Prize winner was imprisoned in 1977 on Robben Island, South Africa?*

A. Nelson Mandela

B. Desmond Tutu

C. Steve Biko

D. Walter Sisulu

277. *Which landmark event took place in 1979 in China, where thousands of students and workers protested for democracy and human rights?*

A. Tiananmen Square Massacre

B. Cultural Revolution

C. Great Leap Forward

D. Democracy Wall Movement

278. *Which European country legalized abortion in 1975, becoming one of the first in the world to do so?*

A. France

B. Sweden

C. Netherlands

D. Italy

279. *Which Middle Eastern country was involved in a hostage crisis in 1979, where 52 American diplomats and citizens were held captive for 444 days?*

A. Iran

B. Iraq

C. Syria

D. Lebanon

280. *Which South American country was ruled by a socialist president who was overthrown by a military coup in 1973?*

A. Chile

B. Argentina

C. Brazil

D. Venezuela

281. *Which personal computer was introduced in 1977 by Apple and became one of the first successful mass-produced microcomputers?*

A. Apple I

B. Apple II

C. Macintosh

D. Lisa

282. *Which genetic engineering technique was developed in 1973 by Stanley Cohen and Herbert Boyer, allowing the transfer of DNA between different organisms?*

A. Polymerase chain reaction

B. DNA sequencing

C. Recombinant DNA

D. Gene therapy

283. *Which space probe was launched in 1977 and carried a golden record with sounds and images of Earth?*

A. Voyager 1

B. Voyager 2

C. Pioneer 10

D. Pioneer 11

284. *Which video game console was released in 1977 by Atari and popularized the use of interchangeable cartridges?*

A. Atari 2600

B. Atari 5200

C. Atari 7800

D. Atari Jaguar

285. *Which scientific theory was proposed in 1974 by Stephen Hawking, suggesting that black holes emit radiation?*

A. Hawking radiation
B. Higgs boson
C. String theory
D. Quantum gravity

286. *Which medical imaging technique was invented in 1971 by Godfrey Hounsfield and Allan Cormack, allowing doctors to see inside the body without surgery?*

A. X-ray
B. MRI
C. CT scan
D. Ultrasound

287. *Which electronic device was invented in 1973 by Martin Cooper and became the first handheld mobile phone?*

A. Motorola DynaTAC
B. Nokia 3310
C. BlackBerry
D. iPhone

288. *Which artificial sweetener was discovered in 1976 by Shashikant Phadnis, who accidentally tasted it while working on an insecticide?*

A. Aspartame
B. Sucralose
C. Saccharin
D. Stevia

289. *Which spacecraft was launched in 1977 and carried a plaque with a message from Earth to any extraterrestrial intelligence?*

A	Voyager 1	B	Voyager 2
C	Pioneer 10	D	Pioneer 11

290. *Which genetic disorder was identified in 1979 by Yuet Wai Kan and Andree Dozy, who found a mutation in the beta-globin gene?*

A	Cystic fibrosis	B	Down syndrome
C	Sickle cell anemia	D	Hemophilia

291. *Which programming language was created in 1972 by Dennis Ritchie and is widely used for system and application development?*

A	C	B	Java
C	Python	D	Pascal

292. *Which nuclear power plant suffered a partial meltdown in 1979, causing a major environmental and health crisis in Pennsylvania?*

A	Chernobyl	B	Fukushima
C	Three Mile Island	D	Sellafield

293. *Which electronic device was invented in 1979 by Sony and allowed people to listen to music on the go?*

A Walkman	B iPod
C Boombox	D CD player

294. *Which Nobel Prize-winning physicist developed the theory of supergravity in 1976, which attempted to unify gravity with other fundamental forces?*

A Albert Einstein	B Stephen Hawking
C Richard Feynman	D Daniel Z. Freedman

295. *Which communication technology was invented in 1973 by Vint Cerf and Bob Kahn, and is the basis of the internet?*

A Ethernet	B Bluetooth
C TCP/IP	D Wi-Fi

296. *Which chemical element was discovered in 1974 by a team of Soviet scientists and named after a Russian physicist?*

A Dubnium	B Seaborgium
C Rutherfordium	D Flerovium

297. *Which optical disc format was invented in 1979 by Philips and Sony and became the standard for storing digital audio?*

A CD

B DVD

C Blu-ray

D LaserDisc

298. *Which branch of mathematics was developed in 1970 by Benoit Mandelbrot, who studied the patterns and shapes of natural phenomena?*

A Chaos theory

B Fractal geometry

C Game theory

D Graph theory

299. *Which medical device was invented in 1978 by Wilson Greatbatch and implanted in a human heart for the first time?*

A Pacemaker

B Stent

C Defibrillator

D Ventilator

300. *Which space shuttle was the first to be launched by NASA in 1977, although it never reached orbit?*

A Columbia

B Challenger

C Discovery

D Enterprise

The 1980's

The Electric 1980s: A Decade of Excess, Innovation, and Iconic Moments

Welcome to the 1980s, an era that turned up the volume on everything from music to fashion to technology. It was a decade of bold styles, neon colors, and unforgettable pop culture moments that have become emblematic of a time when excess was celebrated and innovation was embraced.

The '80s brought us the rise of the personal computer, the thrill of arcade games, and the advent of the music video. It was a time when MTV was born, Michael Jackson reigned as the King of Pop, and Madonna became a cultural icon.

As you dive into the trivia of the 1980s, prepare to be transported back to the days of big hair bands, the Brat Pack, and the fall of the Berlin Wall. This was a decade where the world became smaller through technology, and larger-than-life characters dominated the screen and airwaves.

So grab your leg warmers, pop in a mixtape, and get ready to challenge yourself with memories from the decade that still influences us today. Let's celebrate the 1980s — a time of transformation, imagination, and unforgettable flair!

301. *Which British band had a hit with "Don't You Want Me" in 1981?*

A. The Human League
B. Duran Duran
C. Depeche Mode
D. The Cure

302. *Which American singer won the Grammy Award for Album of the Year in 1984 for "Thriller"?*

A. Michael Jackson
B. Prince
C. Madonna
D. Bruce Springsteen

303. *Which Australian rock band released the album "Back in Black" in 1980, which became one of the best-selling albums of all time?*

A. INXS
B. Men at Work
C. AC/DC
D. Midnight Oil

304. *Which Irish band had their first number-one single in the US with "With or Without You" in 1987?*

A. The Cranberries
B. U2
C. The Pogues
D. The Corrs

305. *Which Swedish pop group won the Eurovision Song Contest in 1984 with the song "Waterloo"?*

A. Roxette
B. ABBA
C. Ace of Base
D. A-ha

306. *Which American rap group released the influential album "Straight Outta Compton" in 1988?*

A. Run-DMC
B. Public Enemy
C. N.W.A
D. Beastie Boys

307. *Which British singer had a hit with "I Want to Break Free" in 1984, which featured a video of him dressed as a woman?*

A. David Bowie
B. Freddie Mercury
C. Rod Stewart
D. Elton John

308. *Which American rock band had their breakthrough album "Appetite for Destruction" in 1987, which included the song "Sweet Child o' Mine"?*

A. Aerosmith
B. Bon Jovi
C. Metallica
D. Guns N' Roses

309. *Which Jamaican singer popularized reggae music in the 1980s with songs like "Red Red Wine" and "I Got You Babe"?*

A) Bob Marley
B) Jimmy Cliff
C) UB40
D) Shaggy

310. *Which Canadian singer won the Eurovision Song Contest in 1988 with the song "Ne partez pas sans moi"?*

A) Celine Dion
B) Shania Twain
C) Alanis Morissette
D) Bryan Adams

311. *Which American singer-songwriter released the album "Graceland" in 1986, which featured collaborations with South African musicians?*

A) Paul Simon
B) Bob Dylan
C) Bruce Springsteen
D) Neil Young

312. *Which British duo had a hit with "West End Girls" in 1985, which topped the charts in both the UK and the US?*

A) Wham!
B) Eurythmics
C) Pet Shop Boys
D) Erasure

313. *Which American pop star had her debut album "Madonna" in 1983, which included the songs "Holiday" and "Lucky Star"?*

A	Madonna	B	Cyndi Lauper
C	Whitney Houston	D	Janet Jackson

314. *Which German band had a hit with "99 Luftballons" in 1983, which was an anti-war protest song?*

A	Kraftwerk	B	Nena
C	Scorpions	D	Rammstein

315. *Which American rock band had their first number-one album in the US with "Slippery When Wet" in 1986, which included the songs "Livin' on a Prayer" and "You Give Love a Bad Name"?*

A	Bon Jovi	B	Aerosmith
C	Guns N' Roses	D	Van Halen

316. *Which American singer had a hit with "Girls Just Want to Have Fun" in 1983, which became an anthem for female empowerment?*

A	Madonna	B	Cyndi Lauper
C	Pat Benatar	D	Tina Turner

317. *Which Scottish band had a hit with "Don't You (Forget About Me)" in 1985, which was featured in the movie "The Breakfast Club"?*

A. Simple Minds
B. The Proclaimers
C. Big Country
D. Deacon Blue

318. *Which American rock band had their first number-one single in the UK with "The Final Countdown" in 1986?*

A. Journey
B. Foreigner
C. Europe
D. Kansas

319. *Which British singer had a hit with "Careless Whisper" in 1984, which was his first solo single after leaving his band?*

A. George Michael
B. Phil Collins
C. Sting
D. David Bowie

320. *Which American pop star had her debut album "Whitney Houston" in 1985, which included the songs "Saving All My Love for You" and "How Will I Know"?*

A. Whitney Houston
B. Mariah Carey
C. Janet Jackson
D. Toni Braxton

321. *Which 1982 movie starred Harrison Ford as a futuristic detective who hunts down rogue androids?*

A   Blade Runner

B   The Terminator

C   RoboCop

D   Total Recall

322. *Which 1984 sitcom featured four older women living together in Miami?*

A   Designing Women

B   The Golden Girls

C   Murphy Brown

D   Cheers

323. *Which 1985 movie was based on a novel by Stephen King and starred Jack Nicholson as a writer who goes insane in a haunted hotel?*

A   The Shining

B   Carrie

C   Misery

D   The Stand

324. *Which 1986 musical drama starred Tom Cruise as a young aspiring rock star who moves to Los Angeles?*

A   Rock of Ages

B   Almost Famous

C   Rock Star

D   Top Gun

325. *Which 1989 animated movie was the first feature film produced by Pixar and featured the voices of Tom Hanks and Tim Allen?*

A. Toy Story
B. A Bug's Life
C. Monsters, Inc.
D. Finding Nemo

326. *Which 1987 movie starred Patrick Swayze and Jennifer Grey as a dance instructor and a shy teenager who fall in love at a resort?*

A. Dirty Dancing
B. Footloose
C. Flashdance
D. Grease

327. *Which 1988 sitcom featured a sarcastic alien who came to live with a suburban family?*

A. Mork & Mindy
B. ALF
C. 3rd Rock from the Sun
D. My Favorite Martian

328. *Which 1981 movie starred Harrison Ford as an adventurous archaeologist who searches for the Ark of the Covenant?*

A. Indiana Jones and the Raiders of the Lost Ark
B. Indiana Jones and the Temple of Doom
C. Indiana Jones and the Last Crusade
D. Indiana Jones and the Kingdom of the Crystal Skull

329. *Which 1983 movie starred Al Pacino as a Cuban refugee who becomes a powerful drug lord in Miami?*

A Scarface

B The Godfather

C Goodfellas

D The Untouchables

330. *Which 1989 animated TV show featured a dysfunctional family of yellow-skinned characters? *

A The Simpsons

B Family Guy

C South Park

D Futurama

331. *Which 1980 movie starred Robert De Niro as a boxer who struggles with his personal and professional life?*

A Raging Bull

B Rocky

C The Fighter

D Million Dollar Baby

332. *Which 1987 TV show featured a team of soldiers of fortune who helped people in need?*

A The A-Team

B MacGyver

C Knight Rider

D Magnum, P.I.

333. *Which 1985 movie starred Michael J. Fox as a teenager who travels back in time to 1955 and meets his parents?*

(A) Back to the Future

(B) The Terminator

(C) Bill & Ted's Excellent Adventure

(D) The Goonies

334. *Which 1982 movie starred Dustin Hoffman as an out-of-work actor who disguises himself as a woman to get a role on a soap opera?*

(A) Tootsie

(B) Mrs. Doubtfire

(C) Some Like It Hot

(D) The Birdcage

335. *Which 1984 movie starred Eddie Murphy as a wisecracking detective who goes to Beverly Hills to investigate a murder?*

(A) Beverly Hills Cop

(B) 48 Hrs.

(C) Lethal Weapon

(D) Die Hard

336. *Which 1980 movie starred Robert De Niro as a boxer who struggles with his personal and professional life?*

(A) Raging Bull

(B) Rocky

(C) The Fighter

(D) Million Dollar Baby

337. *Which 1987 TV show featured a team of soldiers of fortune who helped people in need?*

A	The A-Team	B	MacGyver
C	Knight Rider	D	Magnum, P.I.

338. *Which 1985 movie starred Michael J. Fox as a teenager who travels back in time to 1955 and meets his parents?*

A	Back to the Future	B	The Terminator
C	Bill & Ted's Excellent Adventure	D	The Goonies

339. *Which 1982 movie starred Dustin Hoffman as an out-of-work actor who disguises himself as a woman to get a role on a soap opera?*

A	Tootsie	B	Mrs. Doubtfire
C	Some Like It Hot	D	The Birdcage

340. *Which 1984 movie starred Eddie Murphy as a wisecracking detective who goes to Beverly Hills to investigate a murder?*

A	Beverly Hills Cop	B	48 Hrs.
C	Lethal Weapon	D	Die Hard

341. *Which country hosted the 1980 Summer Olympics, which were boycotted by many Western nations?*

A. China

B. Soviet Union

C. Mexico

D. Canada

342. *Which American boxer became the undisputed heavyweight champion of the world in 1987 by defeating Michael Spinks?*

A. Muhammad Ali

B. Mike Tyson

C. Evander Holyfield

D. George Foreman

343. *Which Italian football club won the European Cup (now Champions League) three times in the 1980s?*

A. Juventus

B. AC Milan

C. Inter Milan

D. Roma

344. *Which Canadian ice hockey player scored 92 goals in the 1981-82 season, setting a new NHL record?*

A. Wayne Gretzky

B. Mario Lemieux

C. Bobby Orr

D. Gordie Howe

345. *Which British athlete won four gold medals at the 1984 and 1988 Summer Olympics in middle-distance running events?*

A	Sebastian Coe	B	Steve Ovett
C	Daley Thompson	D	Steve Cram

346. *Which American basketball player won the NBA Most Valuable Player award five times in the 1980s?*

A	Michael Jordan	B	Magic Johnson
C	Larry Bird	D	Kareem Abdul-Jabbar

347. *Which Argentine footballer scored two famous goals against England in the 1986 World Cup quarter-final, one with his hand and one with his feet?*

A	Diego Maradona	B	Lionel Messi
C	Gabriel Batistuta	D	Mario Kempes

348. *Which Czech tennis player won 18 Grand Slam singles titles in the 1980s, the most of any player in that decade?*

A	Martina Navratilova	B	Steffi Graf
C	Chris Evert	D	Monica Seles

349. *Which American swimmer won seven gold medals at the 1984 Summer Olympics in Los Angeles?*

A. Mark Spitz

B. Michael Phelps

C. Matt Biondi

D. Ryan Lochte

350. *Which British Formula One driver won three world championships in the 1980s, in 1981, 1983, and 1987?*

A. Nigel Mansell

B. Jackie Stewart

C. James Hunt

D. Nelson Piquet

351. *Which American golfer won six major championships in the 1980s, the most of any player in that decade?*

A. Jack Nicklaus

B. Tom Watson

C. Greg Norman

D. Nick Faldo

352. *Which Soviet gymnast won a record nine gold medals at the 1980 and 1988 Summer Olympics?*

A. Olga Korbut

B. Nadia Comaneci

C. Larisa Latynina

D. Nellie Kim

353. *Which New Zealand rugby union team won the first Rugby World Cup in 1987?*

A. All Blacks

B. Wallabies

C. Springboks

D. Lions

354. *Which American baseball player broke the record for most home runs in a single season in 1987 with 49?*

A. Babe Ruth

B. Hank Aaron

C. Mark McGwire

D. Barry Bonds

355. *Which French cyclist won the Tour de France five times in a row from 1981 to 1985?*

A. Jacques Anquetil

B. Bernard Hinault

C. Eddy Merckx

D. Miguel Indurain

356. *Which American football team won four Super Bowls in the 1980s, in 1982, 1985, 1989, and 1990?*

A. Dallas Cowboys

B. San Francisco 49ers

C. Pittsburgh Steelers

D. New York Giants

357. *Which Soviet chess player became the youngest world champion ever in 1985 at the age of 22?*

A. Anatoly Karpov

B. Garry Kasparov

C. Boris Spassky

D. Mikhail Tal

358. *Which Brazilian Formula One driver won his first world championship in 1988, beating his teammate and rival Alain Prost?*

A. Ayrton Senna

B. Nelson Piquet

C. Emerson Fittipaldi

D. Felipe Massa

359. *Which American basketball team won five NBA championships in the 1980s, in 1980, 1982, 1985, 1987, and 1988?*

A. Los Angeles Lakers

B. Boston Celtics

C. Chicago Bulls

D. Detroit Pistons

360. *Which Australian cricket player scored a record 334 runs in a single test match against India in 1980?*

A. Don Bradman

B. Mark Taylor

C. Ricky Ponting

D. Greg Chappell

361. *Which British Prime Minister led the country during the Falklands War in 1982?*

A	Margaret Thatcher	B	John Major
C	Tony Blair	D	Winston Churchill

362. *Which American President was shot and wounded by a would-be assassin in 1981?*

A	Ronald Reagan	B	Jimmy Carter
C	George H. W. Bush	D	Bill Clinton

363. *Which Chinese leader initiated the economic reforms and the open-door policy in the late 1970s and 1980s?*

A	Mao Zedong	B	Deng Xiaoping
C	Jiang Zemin	D	Xi Jinping

364. *Which Polish trade union leader and activist won the Nobel Peace Prize in 1983 for his role in the Solidarity movement?*

A	Lech Walesa	B	Karol Wojtyla
C	Andrzej Duda	D	Adam Michnik

365. *Which South African anti-apartheid leader was released from prison in 1990 after 27 years of incarceration?*

A	Nelson Mandela	B	Desmond Tutu
C	Thabo Mbeki	D	Steve Biko

366. *Which Middle Eastern country was invaded by Iraq in 1990, triggering the Gulf War?*

A	Iran	B	Kuwait
C	Saudi Arabia	D	Syria

367. *Which Soviet leader introduced the policies of glasnost (openness) and perestroika (restructuring) in the mid-1980s?*

A	Leonid Brezhnev	B	Yuri Andropov
C	Mikhail Gorbachev	D	Boris Yeltsin

368. *Which American space shuttle exploded shortly after take-off in 1986, killing all seven crew members on board?*

A	Challenger	B	Columbia
C	Discovery	D	Atlantis

369. *Which British warship was sunk by an Argentine missile during the Falklands War in 1982, killing 20 sailors?*

A. HMS Sheffield

B. HMS Invincible

C. HMS Coventry

D. HMS Exeter

370. *Which Asian country was ruled by the Khmer Rouge regime from 1975 to 1979, which killed millions of people in a genocide?*

A. Vietnam

B. Cambodia

C. Laos

D. Thailand

371. *Which African country was affected by a severe famine in 1984-85, which prompted international relief efforts such as Live Aid?*

A. Ethiopia

B. Somalia

C. Sudan

D. Rwanda

372. *Which American actress and fitness guru was arrested in 1989 for protesting against the Chinese government's crackdown on pro-democracy demonstrators in Tiananmen Square?*

A. Jane Fonda

B. Meryl Streep

C. Cher

D. Susan Sarandon

373. *Which German city was divided by a wall from 1961 to 1989, symbolizing the Cold War between the East and the West?*

A Berlin

B Hamburg

C Munich

D Frankfurt

374. *Which Indian Prime Minister was assassinated by her own bodyguards in 1984, sparking anti-Sikh riots across the country?*

A Indira Gandhi

B Rajiv Gandhi

C Jawaharlal Nehru

D Narendra Modi

375. *Which treaty, signed in 1987, aimed to eliminate intermediate-range nuclear missiles and marked a significant step towards the end of the Cold War?*

A SALT I

B START I

C INF Treaty

D Treaty of Versailles

376. *Which American civil rights leader and Baptist minister ran for the Democratic presidential nomination in 1984 and 1988?*

A Martin Luther King Jr.

B Jesse Jackson

C Malcolm X

D Al Sharpton

377. *Which British rock band performed at the Live Aid concert in 1985 and stole the show with their 20-minute set?*

| A | The Beatles | B | The Rolling Stones |
| C | Queen | D | Led Zeppelin |

378. *Which Asian country was ruled by the dictator Ferdinand Marcos from 1965 to 1986, until he was ousted by a peaceful revolution?*

| A | Philippines | B | Indonesia |
| C | Thailand | D | Malaysia |

379. *Which Middle Eastern country was involved in a long and bloody war with Iran from 1980 to 1988?*

| A | Iraq | B | Syria |
| C | Israel | D | Turkey |

380. *Which American actress and humanitarian was appointed as a Goodwill Ambassador for UNICEF in 1989?*

| A | Audrey Hepburn | B | Marilyn Monroe |
| C | Grace Kelly | D | Elizabeth Taylor |

381. *Which American computer scientist and engineer invented the World Wide Web in 1989?*

A. Tim Berners-Lee
B. Bill Gates
C. Steve Jobs
D. Alan Turing

382. *Which British scientist and author published his best-selling book "A Brief History of Time" in 1988, which explained the origin and structure of the universe?*

A. Isaac Newton
B. Charles Darwin
C. Stephen Hawking
D. Richard Dawkins

383. *Which Japanese company launched the first handheld video game console, the Game Boy, in 1989?*

A. Sony
B. Nintendo
C. Sega
D. Atari

384. *Which American geneticist and Nobel laureate discovered the first human oncogene, a gene that can cause cancer, in 1982?*

A. James Watson
B. Francis Crick
C. Michael Bishop
D. Craig Venter

385: *Which American engineer and inventor developed the first artificial heart, which was implanted in a human patient in 1982?

A. Robert Jarvik

B. Thomas Edison

C. Nikola Tesla

D. Alexander Graham Bell

386. *Which American company introduced the first personal computer with a graphical user interface and a mouse, the Macintosh, in 1984?*

A. IBM

B. Microsoft

C. Apple

D. Dell

387 *Which significant political event in 1989 led to the end of communist rule in Poland and the beginning of the political transformation of Central and Eastern Europe?*

A. The signing of the INF Treaty

B. The fall of the Berlin Wall

C. The Tiananmen Square protests

D. The Round Table Talks

388. *Which American inventor and entrepreneur founded the company NeXT in 1985, after leaving Apple?*

A. Steve Jobs

B. Steve Wozniak

C. Bill Gates

D. Elon Musk

389. *Which environmental disaster in 1986 became the world's worst nuclear accident, leading to significant changes in safety protocols and international policy?*

A. Three Mile Island

B. Fukushima Daiichi

C. Chernobyl

D. Kyshtym Disaster.

390. *Which significant political event in 1989 symbolized the end of the Cold War and led to the reunification of Germany?*

A. The signing of the INF Treaty

B. The election of Ronald Reagan

C. The fall of the Berlin Wall

D. The dissolution of the Soviet Union.

391. *Which American engineer and entrepreneur founded the company Cisco Systems in 1984, which became a leader in networking technology?*

A. Leonard Bosack

B. Steve Jobs

C. Jeff Bezos

D. Mark Zuckerberg

392: *Which American chemist and Nobel laureate discovered the first synthetic gene in 1979, which opened the field of genetic engineering?

A. Linus Pauling

B. Harold Urey

C. Kary Mullis

D. Har Gobind Khorana

393. *Which American company developed the first portable cellular phone, the DynaTAC 8000X, in 1983?*

A	Motorola	B	Nokia
C	Samsung	D	Apple

394. *Which French mathematician and philosopher is considered the father of modern philosophy and coined the famous phrase "I think, therefore I am"?*

A	Ren? Descartes	B	Blaise Pascal
C	Voltaire	D	Jean-Paul Sartre

395. *Which American astronomer and author hosted the popular TV series "Cosmos: A Personal Voyage" in 1980, which explored the mysteries of the universe?*

A	Carl Sagan	B	Neil deGrasse Tyson
C	Stephen Hawking	D	Brian Greene

396. *Which American computer scientist and engineer developed the first web browser, called WorldWideWeb, in 1990?*

A	Tim Berners-Lee	B	Marc Andreessen
C	Robert Cailliau	D	Ted Nelson

397: *Which American physicist and Nobel laureate discovered the first evidence of dark matter in 1980, by studying the rotation of galaxies?

A) Vera Rubin	B) Carl Sagan
C) Edwin Hubble	D) Albert Einstein

398. *Which environmental protocol, signed by nations in 1987, aimed to reduce the production and consumption of substances that deplete the ozone layer?*

A) Kyoto Protocol	B) Montreal Protocol
C) Paris Agreement	D) Rio Declaration.

399. *Which French philosopher and mathematician is considered the father of analytic geometry and the coordinate system, which are named after him?*

A) Ren? Descartes	B) Blaise Pascal
C) Pierre de Fermat	D) Henri Poincar?

400. *Which personal computer, introduced in 1984, featured a graphical user interface and a mouse?*

A) IBM PC	B) Commodore 64
C) Apple Macintosh	D) Amiga 1000

The 1990's

The Transformative 1990s: A Decade of Digital Revolution and Global Connectivity

Embark on a journey back to the 1990s, a pivotal decade that saw the world shrink through the power of the internet and expand with the promise of a new millennium. It was an era of rapid technological advancement, cultural diversity, and political change that reshaped the global landscape.

The '90s were defined by the emergence of grunge music, the dominance of sitcoms like "Friends," and the cinematic wonders of CGI. It was a time when cell phones began to fit in our pockets, gaming consoles battled for supremacy, and the World Wide Web wove its way into daily life.

As you explore the trivia of the 1990s, get ready to relive the excitement of the dot-com boom, the enchantment of "Harry Potter," and the drama of the O.J. Simpson trial. This was a decade where anything seemed possible, and the world tuned in to watch history unfold.

So, rewind your memories, dial-up your spirit of adventure, and let's test your knowledge of the 1990s – a decade that left an indelible mark on the way we live, work, and play. Let the trivia begin!

401. *Which band released the hit song "Smells Like Teen Spirit"?*

A. Nirvana

B. Pearl Jam

C. Red Hot Chili Peppers

D. Metallica

402. *Who was known as the "Queen of Pop" in the 1990s?*

A. Madonna

B. Janet Jackson

C. Mariah Carey

D. Whitney Houston

403. *What was the best-selling album of the 1990s?*

A. "Metallica" by Metallica

B. "Millennium" by Backstreet Boys

C. "Jagged Little Pill" by Alanis Morissette

D. "The Bodyguard" by Whitney Houston

404. *Which group had a hit with "Waterfalls" in 1995?*

A. Destiny's Child

B. TLC

C. Spice Girls

D. No Doubt

405. *Who won the Grammy for Album of the Year in 1999?*

A	Lauryn Hill	B	Shania Twain
C	Madonna	D	Celine Dion

406. *What was the name of Britney Spears' debut single in 1998?*

A	"Oops!... I Did It Again"	B	"Baby One More Time"
C	"Toxic"	D	"Womanizer"

407. *Which band released the album "Nevermind" in 1991?*

A	Green Day	B	Nirvana
C	Soundgarden	D	The Smashing Pumpkins

408. *Who sang the hit "I Will Always Love You" in 1992?*

A	Mariah Carey	B	Toni Braxton
C	Whitney Houston	D	Celine Dion

409. *Which song by the band Oasis became a hit in 1995?*

A	"Live Forever"	**B**	"Champagne Supernova"
C	"Wonderwall"	**D**	"Don't Look Back in Anger"

410. *Who is the lead singer of the band U2?*

A	Bono	**B**	Michael Stipe
C	Chris Martin	**D**	Thom Yorke

411. *Which artist is known for the hit "My Heart Will Go On"?*

A	Mariah Carey	**B**	Shania Twain
C	Celine Dion	**D**	Cher

412. *What was the name of Backstreet Boys' debut album?*

A	"Millennium"	**B**	"Backstreet Boys"
C	"Black & Blue"	**D**	"Backstreet's Back"

413. *Which 1990s song starts with "Today is gonna be the day..."?*

- **A** "Bitter Sweet Symphony" by The Verve
- **B** "Wonderwall" by Oasis
- **C** "Good Riddance" by Green Day
- **D** "Creep" by Radiohead

414. *Who had a hit with "You Oughta Know" in 1995?*

- **A** Fiona Apple
- **B** Alanis Morissette
- **C** Tori Amos
- **D** Sheryl Crow

415. *Which band's debut album was titled "Ten"?*

- **A** Nirvana
- **B** Pearl Jam
- **C** Alice in Chains
- **D** Soundgarden

416. *Which rapper's debut album was "Illmatic"?*

- **A** Jay-Z
- **B** Tupac Shakur
- **C** Notorious B.I.G.
- **D** Nas

417. *What is the title of Spice Girls' debut single?*

A "2 Become 1"

B "Spice Up Your Life"

C "Wannabe"

D "Say You'll Be There"

418. *Which band had a hit with "Losing My Religion" in 1991?*

A R.E.M.

B U2

C Radiohead

D Nirvana

419. *Who released the album "Ray of Light" in 1998?*

A Britney Spears

B Christina Aguilera

C Madonna

D Kylie Minogue

420. *Which song by Coolio featured LV and became a major hit in 1995?*

A "Fantastic Voyage"

B "1, 2, 3, 4 (Sumpin' New)"

C "Gangsta's Paradise"

D "Too Hot"

421. *Which movie featured a young boy who could see dead people?*

A	The Sixth Sense	**B**	Ghost
C	Stir of Echoes	**D**	The Others

422. *What was the name of the main character in "The Matrix"?*

A	Morpheus	**B**	Neo
C	Trinity	**D**	Agent Smith

423. *Who played the lead role in "Forrest Gump"?*

A	Tom Hanks	**B**	Bill Murray
C	Robin Williams	**D**	Jim Carrey

424. *Which sitcom featured the characters Ross, Rachel, and Monica?*

A	Seinfeld	**B**	Friends
C	Frasier	**D**	Will & Grace

425. *What was the highest-grossing film of the 1990s?*

A. Jurassic Park
B. Titanic
C. Star Wars: Episode I – The Phantom Menace
D. Independence Day

426. *Which TV show was set in a bar called Central Perk?*

A. Cheers
B. Friends
C. Frasier
D. The Drew Carey Show

427. *Who directed "Pulp Fiction"?*

A. Steven Spielberg
B. Quentin Tarantino
C. Martin Scorsese
D. Ridley Scott

428. *Which film featured a character named Andy Dufresne?*

A. The Shawshank Redemption
B. The Green Mile
C. Forrest Gump
D. Saving Private Ryan

429. *What was the main profession of the characters in "ER"?*

A. Lawyers

B. Police Officers

C. Doctors

D. Firefighters

430. *Which series followed the investigations of FBI agents Mulder and Scully?*

A. The X-Files

B. Twin Peaks

C. Law & Order

D. NYPD Blue

431. *Which movie introduced the character Jack Dawson?*

A. Good Will Hunting

B. Titanic

C. The Talented Mr. Ripley

D. A Few Good Men

432. *What was the main setting of the TV show "Seinfeld"?*

A. A coffee shop

B. A newsroom

C. An apartment in New York

D. A high school

433. *Who starred as the lead in the movie "Speed"?*

A	Tom Cruise	B	Keanu Reeves
C	Bruce Willis	D	Nicolas Cage

434. *Which TV show's theme song started with the line "I'll be there for you"?*

A	Full House	B	Friends
C	The Fresh Prince of Bel-Air	D	Married... with Children

435. *"Braveheart" won the Academy Award for Best Picture in what year?*

A	1994	B	1995
C	1996	D	1997

436. *Which 1990s movie featured a character named Tyler Durden?*

A	Fight Club	B	American Psycho
C	The Big Lebowski	D	Trainspotting

437. *What was the main setting of the TV show "Friends"?*

A	A coffee shop	B	A bookstore
C	A restaurant	D	An office

438. *Who played the role of Sarah Connor in "Terminator 2: Judgment Day"?*

A	Sigourney Weaver	B	Linda Hamilton
C	Jamie Lee Curtis	D	Geena Davis

439. *Which film won the Oscar for Best Picture in 1999?*

A	The Matrix	B	American Beauty
C	The Sixth Sense	D	Fight Club

440. *Which TV series featured the character George Costanza?*

A	Seinfeld	B	Everybody Loves Raymond
C	King of Queens	D	Friends

441. *Which country hosted the 1992 Summer Olympics?*

A. Spain

B. United States

C. Australia

D. Greece

442. *Who won the FIFA World Cup in 1994?*

A. Italy

B. Brazil

C. Germany

D. Argentina

443. *Which NBA player returned to basketball in 1995 with the phrase "I'm back"?*

A. Magic Johnson

B. Michael Jordan

C. Shaquille O'Neal

D. Larry Bird

444. *What major golf tournament did Tiger Woods win in 1997?*

A. The Open Championship

B. The Masters

C. PGA Championship

D. U.S. Open

445. *Which female tennis player won 22 Grand Slam singles titles in the 1990s?*

A. Martina Navratilova

B. Monica Seles

C. Steffi Graf

D. Serena Williams

446. *Who set the record for most home runs in a single MLB season in 1998?*

A. Mark McGwire

B. Sammy Sosa

C. Ken Griffey Jr.

D. Barry Bonds

447. *Which country won the most gold medals at the 1996 Summer Olympics?*

A. Russia

B. Germany

C. United States

D. China

448. *What was the nickname of NBA player Anfernee Hardaway?*

A. Magic

B. Air

C. Penny

D. The Glove

449. *Which NHL team won the Stanley Cup in 1994?*

(A) Detroit Red Wings

(B) New York Rangers

(C) Montreal Canadiens

(D) Pittsburgh Penguins

450. *Who won the Tour de France four times in the 1990s?*

(A) Lance Armstrong

(B) Greg LeMond

(C) Miguel Indurain

(D) Jan Ullrich

451. *Which figure skater won Olympic gold in 1992 and 1994?*

(A) Nancy Kerrigan

(B) Oksana Baiul

(C) Kristi Yamaguchi

(D) Tonya Harding

452. *What team did Michael Jordan play for after returning from retirement?*

(A) Washington Wizards

(B) Chicago Bulls

(C) Charlotte Hornets

(D) New York Knicks

453. *Which country won the Rugby World Cup in 1995?*

A. New Zealand

B. Australia

C. South Africa

D. England

454. *Who was the first player to be drafted in the 1992 NBA Draft?*

A. Shaquille O'Neal

B. Alonzo Mourning

C. Christian Laettner

D. Jim Jackson

455. *Which female gymnast scored a perfect 10 seven times at the 1992 Olympics?*

A. Shannon Miller

B. Dominique Dawes

C. Lavinia Milo?ovici

D. Svetlana Boginskaya

456. *Which boxer was famously bitten by Mike Tyson during a match?*

A. Lennox Lewis

B. Evander Holyfield

C. Buster Douglas

D. Frank Bruno

457. *What team won the first Premier League title in 1992-93?*

A. Liverpool

B. Arsenal

C. Manchester United

D. Chelsea

458. *Who won the men's singles at Wimbledon in 1990?*

A. Andre Agassi

B. Pete Sampras

C. Boris Becker

D. Stefan Edberg

459. *Which country hosted the Winter Olympics in 1994?*

A. Norway

B. Japan

C. Canada

D. France

460. *Which NFL team won three Super Bowls in the 1990s?*

A. San Francisco 49ers

B. Dallas Cowboys

C. Green Bay Packers

D. Denver Broncos

461. *Which treaty formed the European Union in 1993?*

A. Maastricht Treaty

B. Treaty of Lisbon

C. Treaty of Rome

D. Treaty of Amsterdam

462. *Who became South Africa's first black president in 1994?*

A. Desmond Tutu

B. Thabo Mbeki

C. Nelson Mandela

D. Jacob Zuma

463. *What event marked the end of the Soviet Union in 1991?*

A. The signing of the Belavezha Accords

B. The fall of the Berlin Wall

C. The Chernobyl disaster

D. The launch of Perestroika

464. *Which city was under siege for 1,425 days during the 1990s?*

A. Grozny

B. Sarajevo

C. Dubrovnik

D. Vukovar

465. *What was the name of the operation that began the Gulf War in 1991?*

A. Operation Desert Storm

B. Operation Iraqi Freedom

C. Operation Enduring Freedom

D. Operation Just Cause

466. *Which peace agreement was signed in 1998 in Northern Ireland?*

A. Belfast Agreement

B. Dublin Agreement

C. Good Friday Agreement

D. Easter Monday Agreement

467. *Who was the Russian president after Boris Yeltsin's resignation in 1999?*

A. Dmitry Medvedev

B. Vladimir Putin

C. Mikhail Gorbachev

D. Viktor Chernomyrdin

468. *What was the international treaty that aimed to reduce greenhouse gas emissions, adopted in 1997?*

A. Paris Agreement

B. Kyoto Protocol

C. Montreal Protocol

D. Stockholm Convention

469. *Which two countries reunited in 1990?*

A. North and South Vietnam

B. East and West Germany

C. North and South Yemen

D. Czech Republic and Slovakia

470. *What major event occurred on September 4, 1998, in the tech industry?*

A. Launch of Windows 98

B. Founding of Google

C. Introduction of the first iMac

D. Release of the Nokia 5110

471. *Which spacecraft was launched by NASA in 1990 to observe distant galaxies?*

A. Voyager 2

B. Hubble Space Telescope

C. Galileo

D. Cassini

472. *Who was the Prime Minister of the UK for most of the 1990s?*

A. Margaret Thatcher

B. Tony Blair

C. John Major

D. Gordon Brown

473. *What was the main currency in Russia before the ruble stabilization of 1998?*

A) Soviet ruble

B) Russian ruble

C) Kopek

D) Denga

474. *Which historic agreement was signed by Israel and Palestine in 1993?*

A) Camp David Accords

B) Oslo Accords

C) Wye River Memorandum

D) Road Map for Peace

475. *What was the popular name for the economic crisis that hit Asia in 1997?*

A) The Great Depression

B) Black Monday

C) The Asian Financial Crisis

D) The Dotcom Bubble

476. *Which U.S. President was impeached in 1998?*

A) George H.W. Bush

B) Bill Clinton

C) George W. Bush

D) Ronald Reagan

477. *What was the name of the sheep that was the first mammal cloned from an adult somatic cell?*

A. Molly
B. Dolly
C. Polly
D. Holly

478. *Which city hosted the 1996 Summer Olympics?*

A. Atlanta
B. Sydney
C. Barcelona
D. Beijing

479. *Who was awarded the Nobel Peace Prize in 1993 alongside Nelson Mandela?*

A. Desmond Tutu
B. F.W. de Klerk
C. Yitzhak Rabin
D. Shimon Peres

480. *What was the major global concern that led to widespread panic as the year 2000 approached?*

A. Global Warming
B. Y2K Bug
C. Dotcom Bubble Burst
D. Ozone Layer Depletion

481. *Which planet was discovered to have ice caps in 1999?*

A	Venus	B	Mars
C	Jupiter	D	Saturn

482. *What was the first cloned animal, born in 1996?*

A	Sheep	B	Mouse
C	Cow	D	Goat

483. *Who developed the World Wide Web in 1990?*

A	Bill Gates	B	Steve Jobs
C	Tim Berners-Lee	D	Linus Torvalds

484. *What significant medical device was first introduced in 1998?*

A	Artificial Heart	B	Portable Ultrasound
C	Viagra	D	Cochlear Implant

485. *Which space telescope was launched into orbit in 1990?*

A	James Webb Space Telescope	B	Spitzer Space Telescope
C	Hubble Space Telescope	D	Chandra X-ray Observatory

486. *What innovation in computer technology was released by IBM in 1997?*

A	The first smartphone	B	The first tablet
C	Deep Blue, the chess-playing computer	D	The USB flash drive

487. *Which mammal was the first to be successfully cloned from an adult cell in 1996?*

A	Mouse	B	Sheep
C	Cow	D	Pig

488. *What was the name of the first rover to land on Mars in 1997?*

A	Curiosity	B	Opportunity
C	Sojourner	D	Spirit

489. *Which company introduced the first commercial MP3 player in 1998?*

A. Sony

B. Apple

C. SaeHan Information Systems

D. Philips

490. *What was the significant breakthrough in human genome mapping announced in 1999?*

A. Completion of the Human Genome Project

B. Discovery of CRISPR

C. First draft sequence of the human genome

D. Cloning of the first human embryo

491. *Which company released the first version of Java in 1995?*

A. Microsoft

B. Apple

C. Sun Microsystems

D. IBM

492. *What was the first animal to be cloned from an adult somatic cell, announced in 1997?*

A. Rat

B. Sheep

C. Rabbit

D. Frog

493. *Which space mission successfully deployed the Galileo spacecraft into Jupiter's orbit in 1995?*

A. Voyager 2
B. Cassini-Huygens
C. Galileo
D. New Horizons

494. *What revolutionary product did Sony introduce in 1994 that changed the gaming industry?*

A. PlayStation
B. Xbox
C. Game Boy Color
D. Sega Saturn

495. *Which medical breakthrough in gene therapy was achieved in 1990?*

A. First successful gene therapy on humans
B. Discovery of the BRCA1 gene
C. Cloning of Dolly the sheep
D. Introduction of antiretroviral therapy for HIV

496. *Which internet browser was introduced by Microsoft in 1995?*

A. Netscape Navigator
B. Internet Explorer
C. Mozilla Firefox
D. Opera

497. *What was the first successfully cloned mammal, announced in 1996?*

A. Cat
B. Sheep
C. Dog
D. Mouse

498. *Which company released Windows 95, a major advancement in PC operating systems?*

A. Apple
B. IBM
C. Microsoft
D. Linux

499. *What significant event in space exploration occurred on July 4, 1997?*

A. The Pathfinder spacecraft landed on Mars
B. The International Space Station was launched
C. The first space tourist traveled to space
D. The Cassini spacecraft was launched to Saturn

500. *Which innovation in communication was released by Nokia in 1992?*

A. The first color mobile phone
B. The first camera mobile phone
C. The first GSM mobile phone
D. The first smartphone

Answers for 1950's

Q	A		Q	A		Q	A		Q	A	
1	B		26	A		51	A		76	D	
2	B		27	D		52	C		77	C	
3	D		28	B		53	B		78	B	
4	C		29	C		54	B		79	B	
5	C		30	B		55	D		80	D	
6	A		31	A		56	D		81	A	
7	B		32	C		57	C		82	A	
8	B		33	B		58	C		83	B	
9	A		34	B		59	B		84	A	
10	B		35	B		60	C		85	D	
11	A		36	A		61	B		86	B	
12	C		37	A		62	C		87	A	
13	B		38	A		63	B		88	C	
14	C		39	A		64	B		89	B	
15	C		40	B		65	B		90	B	
16	A		41	C		66	A		91	B	
17	B		42	B		67	C		92	D	
18	C		43	C		68	B		93	B	
19	A		44	D		69	C		94	B	
20	B		45	C		70	B		95	B	
21	A		46	B		71	D		96	C	
22	C		47	B		72	C		97	B	
23	B		48	C		73	B		98	C	
24	C		49	B		74	A		99	C	
25	B		50	B		75	B		100	C	

Answers for 1960's

Q	A		Q	A		Q	A		Q	A
101	C		126	C		151	D		176	B
102	B		127	B		152	B		177	B
103	B		128	C		153	B		178	C
104	A		129	B		154	A		179	B
105	C		130	B		155	C		180	B
106	A		131	B		156	D		181	B
107	B		132	B		157	B		182	A
108	C		133	C		158	A		183	B
109	A		134	B		159	B		184	A
110	A		135	A		160	B		185	C
111	A		136	A		161	B		186	A
112	B		137	C		162	D		187	B
113	A		138	B		163	A		188	B
114	D		139	C		164	C		189	B
115	A		140	C		165	C		190	C
116	B		141	C		166	B		191	A
117	B		142	B		167	B		192	B
118	C		143	A		168	C		193	C
119	C		144	A		169	B		194	B
120	C		145	B		170	C		195	C
121	C		146	B		171	A		196	B
122	A		147	C		172	A		197	A
123	B		148	B		173	B		198	B
124	A		149	C		174	C		199	B
125	B		150	B		175	C		200	B

Answers for 1970's

Q	A		Q	A		Q	A		Q	A	
201	A		226	A		251	A		276	A	
202	A		227	A		252	D		277	D	
203	B		228	A		253	C		278	A	
204	A		229	C		254	B		279	A	
205	A		230	D		255	A		280	A	
206	A		231	A		256	D		281	B	
207	A		232	A		257	A		282	C	
208	A		233	A		258	A		283	A	
209	C		234	D		259	A		284	A	
210	A		235	A		260	B		285	A	
211	C		236	A		261	A		286	C	
212	A		237	B		262	C		287	A	
213	A		238	A		263	C		288	B	
214	B		239	D		264	D		289	C	
215	A		240	C		265	A		290	C	
216	A		241	A		266	B		291	A	
217	A		242	A		267	D		292	C	
218	C		243	B		268	A		293	A	
219	B		244	B		269	C		294	D	
220	A		245	A		270	B		295	C	
221	A		246	D		271	B		296	D	
222	B		247	B		272	A		297	A	
223	A		248	B		273	C		298	B	
224	C		249	B		274	C		299	A	
225	C		250	A		275	C		300	D	

Answers for 1980's

Q	A		Q	A		Q	A		Q	A	
301	A		326	A		351	B		376	B	
302	A		327	B		352	D		377	C	
303	C		328	A		353	A		378	A	
304	B		329	A		354	C		379	A	
305	B		330	A		355	B		380	A	
306	C		331	A		356	B		381	A	
307	B		332	A		357	B		382	C	
308	D		333	A		358	A		383	B	
309	C		334	A		359	A		384	C	
310	A		335	A		360	D		385	A	
311	A		336	A		361	A		386	C	
312	C		337	A		362	A		387	D	
313	A		338	A		363	B		388	A	
314	B		339	A		364	A		389	C	
315	A		340	A		365	A		390	C	
316	B		341	B		366	B		391	A	
317	A		342	B		367	C		392	D	
318	C		343	B		368	A		393	A	
319	A		344	A		369	A		394	A	
320	A		345	D		370	B		395	A	
321	A		346	C		371	A		396	D	
322	B		347	A		372	A		397	A	
323	A		348	A		373	A		398	B	
324	D		349	C		374	A		399	A	
325	A		350	D		375	C		400	B	

Answers for 1990's

Q	A		Q	A		Q	A		Q	A	
401	A		426	B		451	C		476	B	
402	A		427	B		452	B		477	B	
403	D		428	A		453	C		478	A	
404	B		429	C		454	A		479	B	
405	A		430	A		455	C		480	B	
406	B		431	B		456	B		481	B	
407	B		432	C		457	C		482	A	
408	C		433	B		458	C		483	C	
409	C		434	B		459	A		484	C	
410	A		435	B		460	B		485	C	
411	C		436	A		461	A		486	C	
412	B		437	A		462	C		487	B	
413	B		438	B		463	A		488	C	
414	B		439	B		464	B		489	C	
415	B		440	A		465	A		490	C	
416	D		441	A		466	A		491	C	
417	C		442	B		467	B		492	B	
418	A		443	B		468	B		493	C	
419	C		444	B		469	B		494	A	
420	C		445	C		470	B		495	A	
421	A		446	A		471	B		496	B	
422	B		447	C		472	C		497	B	
423	A		448	C		473	B		498	C	
424	B		449	B		474	B		499	A	
425	B		450	C		475	C		500	C	

www.ingramcontent.com/pod-product-compliance
Lightning Source LLC
Chambersburg PA
CBHW071021250726
48653CB00005B/1674